The 48 Hour Diet

Intermittent Fasting for Healthy, Permanent Weight Loss

I0411348

Margaret Mackenzie

© 2013 by Margaret Mackenzie

ISBN-13: 978-1482706659
ISBN-10: 1482706652

Weight Loss Disclaimer

This book contains weight loss strategies and other health advice that, regardless of my own results and experience, may not produce the same results (or any results) for you. I, or my publishers, make absolutely no guarantee, expressed or implied, that by following the advice below you will lose any weight or improve your health in any way, as there are many factors and variables that come into play regarding any given diet. Any and all weight loss mentioned in this book should be considered as the author's personal experience only and your weight loss potential should be taken on an individual basis, there are too many variables and factors for the values in this book to be considered as what you may be able to lose.

Liability Disclaimer

By reading this book, you assume all risks associated with using the advice given below, with a full understanding that you, solely, are responsible for anything that may occur as a result of putting this information into action in any way, and regardless of your interpretation of the advice.

You further agree that our company cannot be held responsible in any way for the success or failure of your activities as a result of the information presented in this book. It is your responsibility to conduct your own due diligence regarding the safe and successful execution of your diet and lifestyle if you intend to apply any of our information in any way to your situation.

To the fullest extent permitted by law, the sellers are providing this written material, its subsidiary elements and its contents on an 'as is' basis and make no (and expressly disclaim all) representations or warranties of any kind with respect to this material or its contents including, without limitation, advice and recommendations, warranties or merchantability and fitness for a particular purpose. The information is given for entertainment purposes only. In addition, we do not represent or warrant that the information accessible via this material is accurate, complete or current. To the fullest extent permitted by law, neither the sellers or any of its affiliates, partners, directors, employees or other representatives will be liable for damages arising out of or in connection with the use of this material. This is a comprehensive limitation of liability that applies to all damages of any kind, including (without limitation) compensatory, direct, indirect or consequential damages, loss of data, income or profit, loss of or damage to property, damage to health and well being and claims of third parties. This volume is sold for entertainment purposes only, and the author, publishers and/or distributors are not responsible for any actions taken as a result of reading this course.

Terms of Use

You are given a non-transferable, "personal use" license to this book. You cannot distribute it or share it with other individuals.

Also, there are no resale rights or private label rights granted when purchasing this book. In other words, it's for your own personal use only.

Trademarks

Any and all trademarks, either written or shown in pictures, are the property of the respective trademark owners.

The 48 Hour Diet

Intermittent Fasting for Healthy, Permanent Weight Loss

Table of Contents

Highlights

- Lose weight
- Significantly reduce your risk of type 2 diabetes
- Lower your blood pressure
- Reduce cancer risks
- Maybe even reduce your risk of alzheimers

2 Comforting facts

1) Fasting does not mean total abstention from food on fast days.

2) 500 calories is more food than you think.

Publisher's note:

We have included approximate imperial measures after metric measures are given, for the benefit of US readers and also where known language differences exist. We may not know or notice all language differences between English and American but we hope we've managed to get them all. Where clothing sizes are mentioned they're in UK dress sizes, we have attempted to offer US and EU equivalents but there doesn't seem to be a definitive conversion available, find 5 different guides and you'll find 5 different answers. We've used what we believe are the most accurate conversions but there could be errors with them.

Chapter 1. The diet and me

As this is a personal account I had better tell you a little about myself. I am retired and live in Scotland on the banks of the River Forth just North of Edinburgh. I have always been well built and years ago I started to eat more sensibly, mainly by cutting out desserts except on special occasions like birthdays or when I was visiting. Picky guests can be very irritating! I also cut out a lot of obviously fatty food like pastry and some meat products. Despite this the weight slowly crept on and I was a size 22 (US 18, EU 50), verging on 24 (US 20, EU 52) when the doctor suggested that I might be at risk from type 2 diabetes. It was obviously time to do something more drastic. In the distant past I had tried calorie counting and I had been to a weight loss club. I found that these methods didn't work for me because they focused on food. I was thinking about food all the time in a negative way. It was all about the things I shouldn't eat. I felt deprived when I was told that cheese had far too many calories to eat if you wanted to lose weight. A lifetime without my favourite food was a depressing thought. It seemed to me that dieting would have to be for life not only because I had a lot of weight to lose but most of the people I knew who successfully lost weight then gradually put it all back on again, and quite often extra too.

As I had never lost more than a few pounds without a lot of effort I couldn't imagine being thin without permanent and severe deprivation. I was a bit more strict about not eating sweet foods and that was that until I saw a programme on the television. It was about having a very low calorie intake to lower the level of glucose in the blood and so having a lower diabetes risk. It is evidently only necessary to have the very low intake for a short time, fairly frequently. I thought straight away that this was something that I could probably do. It seemed to be a positive way forwards. After all everyone can give up their favourite foods for just one day.

The basic idea is that you have 500 calories (600 for a man) on two days a week and lots to drink. Your body burns calories. After a day or so on a very low intake it is thought that the body believes that a period of famine may be about to start so it slows down its calorie use. Extra fasting is therefore counter productive. In this case more is definitely not better. On the other five days you eat normally. You can eat anything you like. I still kept an eye on what I ate as I have a lot of weight to lose. There seems to be no point at all in blowing your effort on fast days by binging on the other days. However if I feel a desperate craving for my favourite food then I have it without feeling guilty. I find that it's very helpful on fast days to be able to tell myself – "I can't have that today but if I still really want it I can have it tomorrow". Usually by the next day I realised that I didn't want it that much after all and often I had forgotten all about it.

You will lose weight on this regime as long as you are sensible. I have lost one and a half dress sizes over five months (which included a week's holiday over Christmas). I have achieved this steady weight loss without feeling deprived, without thinking about food too much and without getting the baggy skin that goes with rapid weight loss. The best thing is that I feel that I can continue with this way of eating for as long as I need to. There is no boast of loss in pounds and ounces as I gave up scales long ago but I can wear clothes that have been packed away for years. That means more to me than numbers on a scale.

If you have a lot of weight to lose don't expect your friends to notice a difference for quite some time. You and your close family will notice but I am still waiting for friends to see the difference and I expect your friends will be much the same. I have chosen not to tell people about my change in eating habits as I find all the diet talk that follows is very tedious. They will eventually see for themselves!

Chapter 2. Life giving health benefits apart from weight loss?

As I had been warned by my doctor that I was at risk I was very interested in the claims that fasting would significantly lower my chances of developing diabetes. When I discovered that diabetes is connected to a considerably increased risk of heart disease, stroke, blindness and poor circulation resulting in amputation of hands or feet (the increased risk of impotence is probably of more direct importance to male readers) I felt it was worth a big effort to avoid all this suffering. You may be able to take tablets to help your body cope with this condition but what would your quality of life be like?

When we eat sugars and starches the body turns them into glucose to use as fuel which enters the blood stream. To regulate the level of glucose in the blood the pancreas makes insulin. If you have very high levels of glucose the insulin levels in your body can't just go on rising to keep up with the glucose. As the cells in your body become resistant to insulin your glucose levels will stay high. You now have diabetes.

One way you can buy a return ticket for the trip back down this track before you reach the final station is to try intermittent fasting. It is known to work for a lot of people but I am not sure if anyone knows exactly why it works yet. I didn't want to wait until theory caught up with experience - it might have been too late by then.

Fasting is thought to lower the levels of low-density lipoprotein, often called "bad cholesterol", in the blood. This has to be good news.

You may also decrease your risk of cancer (I am looking forward to finding out more about this in the book that Dr Mosley has just published. I have a copy on order. There are details on the last page in case you would like to do the same).

There are suggestions that intermittent fasting can help to combat Alzheimer's disease, dementia and memory loss. The theory is that fasting causes new nerve connections to develop in the brain because in a time of famine the people who have good memories and the ability to think things through have the best chance of survival. So far I believe this is still in the experimental stage and not actually proven but at my age I don't have time to wait around for absolute proof. I dread turning into an animated vegetable, a drag on my family and a drain on resources so I would fast for this benefit alone in the hope that the theory is right.

If this way of eating, or rather not eating, which is already delivering weight loss, can give these extra benefits I feel that I am winning all ways round. It is a big incentive to keep on fasting.

If you are interested in the studies that form the basis of this diet go to www.thefastdiet.co.uk

Chapter 3. Give it a try

Now you know a little about the diet, how do you feel about giving it a try? If you feel like me about traditional dieting and have no patience with fad diets then this might be for you.

A day without food sounds a bit scary. It is a step into the unknown for most of us but there is nothing to be afraid of. One of the very early things I experienced was a feeling of lightness – not physical weight loss but a lightness of spirit. It was good and it is still with me although not as intensely now.

It is a very simple regime which does not dominate your life and it really does work. If you want to go ahead I would like you to have the benefit of some of the things I have learnt along the way.

The **main** thing I discovered was that hunger does not start and then just carry on getting worse and worse. It goes away but may come back later. I found that keeping busy, preferably with things I enjoy doing, was very good for keeping the hunger pangs on the run. By "keeping busy" I don't mean that I was rushing round doing things all the time. Keeping your mind busy works just as well. You should welcome a certain level of hunger as it shows that your diet is working.

The other important thing I found out was that 500 calories can be quite a big meal if you choose carefully (600 for a man).

Choose the days you will fast with care. They should fit into your life with the least possible disruption. Fast on the same days each week. It is now believed that the fast days don't have to be consecutive so choose days that are the most convenient for you as the fasting has to fit into your life or you will abandon it. If you fast on the same days each week it becomes a habit that you don't have to think about. I find

Monday and Tuesday suit me best as I tend to be busier later in the week. I now know that I never have breakfast on Mondays so I don't just go into my morning routine and eat breakfast by mistake. As you can probably tell I am not a morning person and I tend to work on automatic for the first hour or two. If you fast on consecutive days you will find the second day a little more difficult but not as much as you might imagine. I am certainly ready for my bowl of porridge on Wednesday morning! At the moment I am considering splitting the fast days as I now have more commitments on Tuesdays. If I eat at mid-day before I go out I am really hungry by bedtime, especially as I have been fasting on Monday. There is no virtue in making it harder than it needs to be.

The next thing to choose is the time or times when you will eat. I had to experiment for several weeks before I discovered what suited me best. I wake up feeling quite hungry so it seemed like a good idea to start the day with a meal but I was really hungry by bedtime and very tempted to eat sweet sugary things. The up side is that you sleep through the last hours of your fast and there is no will power needed then unless you suffer from insomnia. You have a meal when you get up to fuel you for the day ahead. This might work well for those people who go out to work.

Next I tried having a meal at lunch time and this worked reasonably well although I was still feeling in need of a snack in the evening. The evening is a danger time for me as I am a nibbler. I will have a few nuts, a slice off the block of cheese, a biscuit (cookie) or two... This is especially so when I am on my own. To cut down the temptation I started to eat in the early evening, about 6pm, but by then I was tempted to pile more than 500 calories worth of food onto my plate.

The ideal time for me to eat proved to be about 3:30pm most days. If I'm going to be out all afternoon, especially if I'm going to be reasonably active, then I eat before I go. Common sense and flexibility help you stick to your eating plan. As we all have different metabolisms and different life styles the timing of your meal is something to work out for yourself.

When I first came across the fast diet I understood that it was best to have all the calories at one meal but now it seems that it works just as well if you split the allowance and have a small breakfast and then a slightly larger meal later in the day. This is probably a more sensible routine if you are going out to work. You could use your lunch hour to do something you would enjoy. Personally I would not go shopping as my resistance to snack foods is low if I am at all hungry. I decided not to split my allowance into two meals because I am tempted to snack while preparing my meal. It is easier for me to resist once rather than twice.

Eating in the afternoon has an unexpected benefit for me. It means that I can stay out of the kitchen for most of the day. When I am in the kitchen I snack without thinking. Several times I have had something half way to my mouth before realising that I shouldn't be eating it! On fasting days my husband looks after himself and this has a good spin off. He is learning to cook. Previous suggestions that cookery would be a good thing to learn have been seed scattered on stony ground. Now, to help me, he is having a go and actually quite enjoying the results. It is much easier if you are not around food and I don't think I would have done as well if I had still been cooking for a family. I have always cooked from basic ingredients and there are many opportunities to nibble along the way. This is quite old fashioned, I realise, and many families now live on ready prepared meals that just need putting into the microwave or oven. There are fewer opportunities to snack when preparing this sort of meal. Staying out of temptation makes sense for most of us. There is no merit, or any extra benefit, to be gained by making it any harder for yourself than it needs to be.

Obviously I think most about food at times when I would normally be eating and I find it is much better to be occupied then. I treat myself to time in my sewing room so that Mondays and Tuesdays are days that I look forward to as well as being fast days. I enjoy creative fabric work and show work in exhibitions. Taking time for something I enjoy makes the days a positive experience rather than just a "doing without day".

For me there are psychological elements in keeping the fast. I know that if I break the fast, even by a biscuit's (cookie's) worth, it will be much easier to do the same next time I feel a little peckish. Crossing the barrier of no food except at your meals would be the start of a slippery slope for me. Being aware of that helps me to resist and after all it is only until tomorrow. Not for always.

Now we arrive at the burning question. What should I eat? Again that really depends on your individual tastes to some extent. It is better not to eat a lot of carbohydrate. I find this a deprivation as I feel as if I haven't eaten if the meal has no element of carbohydrate. However you could, for example, have:

2 rashers of lean bacon (fat cut off), grilled with 4 cherry tomatoes (halved) and topped with a poached egg and even add a bunch of watercress for about 270 calories.

Or

Salmon (150g (5 1/4 oz) piece) baked in foil with a big portion of steamed vegetables and a very small portion of plain rice for about 450 calories.

Or

For 350 calories – 2 eggs scrambled in 15g (1/2 oz) of butter (a non stick pan helps) with about 75g (2 1/2 oz) of smoked salmon served on a slice of toast from a small loaf. Add herbs to the scramble for extra taste and use the smoked salmon pieces rather than the whole slices for a more economical dish.

Or

Cottage pie using very low fat minced beef or minced turkey which is a lot cheaper and has next to no fat. Add vegetables to bulk out the meat – celery, leek, carrots and tinned tomatoes. You can also use a stock cube and tomato purée. Top with boiled, mashed potatoes. Use milk or crème fresh for the mashing rather than butter. This will cost you about 450 calories for a small to medium portion.

All these examples could be served to a family. If you do this you will have to be strict with yourself about portion size. I know that gradually, over time, I would take a little more and then a little more still until I would be eating a large portion. It is better for me to have a meal that I create on a plate with the portion size determined before I start. As it's only for two days a week it's no trouble making a separate meal especially as now my husband will make his own!

Chapter 4. The food - what do I eat?

I treat myself to things that I like. If I am only eating once a day I want to enjoy the food. That is why I always lay the table and make it into an occasion. I want to concentrate on enjoying the meal so, while I may listen to the radio, I do not watch television, read or do crosswords. If I do other things the food goes down without me noticing it much and I am left feeling that I haven't had very much at all.

Today I shall have cold roast chicken with a plate heaped up with raw vegetables – carrot, celery, lettuce, cherry tomatoes, cauliflower and slices of an orange bell pepper. This is what I happen to have in the fridge. With that I shall have 2 oatcakes (the Scottish kind that are crispy and about two and a half inches across) and maybe the thinnest sliver of cheese on them.

My meal often follows this basic pattern. I like raw vegetables and they have a variety of texture as well as taste. The protein element changes from day to day and is quite often fish either fresh or canned. I always try to make sure it's fairly low fat protein to keep more calories for other things. I get plenty of fat on other days! I could put all the vegetables in a blender and make a smoothie. It would have the same nutritional value both vitamins, minerals and calories but it would be gone in a matter of minutes. I feel that the time and effort taken to chew the food also helps me to feel fuller. At the most basic level all the chewed bits of fibre and food will take up more room in my stomach and will take longer to digest so I feel fuller for longer. The only drawback I have found with this diet is that I have developed a tendency to be constipated. I prefer the fibre in an unprocessed state to encourage my digestive system to keep on working. Fruit is good too but it has a higher calorie count because of the sugar content.

I sometimes have an omelette and discover from the "Hairy Bikers Cook Book"[1] that I could have a 3 egg omelette with 100g (3 1/2 oz) of prawns in it for 400 calories. I would have to cook in a non stick pan with minimal oil. I could vary the filling although perhaps not cheese. With the spare 100 calories you could have a grilled tomato and a slice of Ryvita – a low calorie crispbread. This does not sound so penitential does it? Fasting conjurers up visions of bread and water not a feast like this.

Scrambled eggs or a Spanish omelette are good too and you can always have a little salad on the side. Once you get going there are a wide variety of thing to choose from. You need never have boring meals.

If the weather is cold I have found that a small portion of soup to start the meal is very comforting. I usually make my own soup as canned soups can contain a very high level of fat and sugar. A simple vegetable soup with no thickening made with good stock from which any fat has been skimmed is ideal. French onion soup is also good. Cream soups, or broths containing pulses (e.g. Scotch Broth which contains barley, lentils and split peas) would take a big chunk from your daily allowance.

---

1 I have found some good ideas for meals in the book by Dave Myers and Si King otherwise known as the "Hairy Bikers". They are cooks and motor bikers who are also big eaters. This book contains calorie counted recipes as they both needed to tackle a spiralling weight problem.

The Hairy Dieters by Dave Myers and Si King
Published by Orion
ISBN 978-1-407-23986-6

To sum up:

- Cook using the absolute minimum of oil or fat. Olive oil has exactly the same number of calories as any other oil. It is not magic in this respect!

- If you are eating food from cans or packets or pre-prepared food of any kind check the calorie content. You may get some big surprises. I know I did. For example savoury crackers with a high sugar content.

- Watch the portion size like a hawk. It can easily increase without you realising what is happening.

- If you "cheat" on the calorie count the only person you are cheating is yourself – and no one is forcing you to do this.

- Find food that you enjoy and eat a variety of things.

- This meal is special so make an occasion of it.

- It is worth a little effort to make your meal interesting as you have a lot to gain from sticking with this diet for the long term.

- Be flexible in your approach to when and what you eat so that this new way of eating fits into your lifestyle.

- Remember it is working for me and it will work for you if you put in the effort.

Chapter 5. The drinks

It is important to maintain your body fluid level while you are fasting. You feel dreadful if you dehydrate and it's quite easy to become dehydrated if you're not aware of the danger. Apart from that I found that drinking helped me over the hunger pangs. I have coffee or tea with skimmed milk three or four times a day. Bearing in mind that milk adds to the calorie count I have water, red bush tea or green tea at other times. I find it easier to drink water if it is hot but that is just a personal preference and probably a lot to do with the climate here. If I feel really hungry I find that a drink with milk in it is much more satisfying. Fruit juice contains sugar so I avoid it on fast days.

Alcohol is just too high in calories for a fast day. It's so high in calories that there would be very little of the allowance left over for food! If I want an alcoholic drink on non-fast days I tend to choose the lower alcohol drinks as these are less fattening (although obviously not some of the hideously sweet concoctions that are on sale these days). This applies mainly to wines and beers. Spirits are high in alcohol and therefore calories but, for most people on this diet, it is quality rather than quantity that counts. Spirits are usually only drunk in small amounts. In a pub (bar) the spirit measures are small so that makes it easy to restrict intake. You can use the same size measures at home as well. Because alcoholic drinks are so high in calories it is important to moderate your intake.

The UK government department of health suggests that two days a week without alcohol gives your liver a rest so the fast diet could help your general health in this way as well.

Chapter 6. The rest of the week

If you are thin and just following this regime for the health benefits or only want to lose a stone (14 pounds) or so then you just carry on in your normal way for the rest of the week. Skip the rest of this chapter, apart from the "treats" section.

Treats

Give yourself treats. They help you along. When that waistband fastens without having to breathe in and without stretching the fabric you have taken a big step on the road and it's an achievement to celebrate. I do **not** choose food related treats. After all you can eat a favourite thing on non fasting days. I prefer a bunch of flowers, a plant for the garden, a visit to an interesting place, a bottle of perfume etc. Not clothes as I don't intend to stay this size for more than a few months to wear them. When the measuring tape shows another inch off your waist measurement have a celebration. You have achieved another step along the way.

Treats are especially important if you have a long way to go. I expect to take about 18 months to lose 3 UK dress sizes. A few treats along the way to celebrate progress will be very welcome. I have not been setting goals as I don't want the pressure that comes with that but once I have reached a point that I decide deserves a treat I then choose a reward. When I dropped a dress size I celebrated by buying some beautiful, but rather expensive, sewing threads. Every time I use them I am reminded of a success and feel good.

Normal eating for big eaters

Those of us who need to lose a lot of weight might well have to be more cautious in responding to the "eat as normal" instruction. Our version of normal eating is what has put us in this position to start with. If we were not "big eaters" then we wouldn't be so fat. I know that if I were to eat as I used to before I took steps to try and stop my weight increasing I could easily make up a lot of the 3000 calories that I save by fasting on the five "eat what you please" days. Having made the effort to fast I do not want to throw away the benefits so eating normally for me has to be eating as I have for the last five years.

It is important not to "make up" for the fast days on the other 5. That defeats the whole object of the exercise.

You will make your own decisions about what would be best for you but I will tell you what has become normal for me. It is not set in stone and I do sometimes have an ice cream or a chocolate bar without feeling bad about it. I sometimes eat lasagne or fish and chips but not too often. The way I eat has become a habit and an attitude of mind so I don't usually think about it much.

It is still worthwhile fasting even if you are eating large very high calorie meals and snacks on the normal days. There are still two days a week when you only have 500 calories of meals. You might find that you actually feel less hungry on the normal days. You will still lose weight and remember the diet is not only about weight loss but about important health benefits as well.

The best thing I did was to decrease my portion size. It was quite difficult to begin with and I don't eat tiny portions now but they are smaller than they used to be.

I gave up full fat milk and now use skimmed for everything. I prefer fresh milk, not the powdered kind. When you first change the milk tastes very thin but you soon get used to it and now I find the full fat milk too greasy. Do **not** give skimmed milk to young children as they need the fat to help them grow. I think we all need the calcium that milk supplies as so many people that I know are suffering from osteoporosis (thinning of the bones). If you find skimmed milk too hard to get used to try switching to semi-skimmed for a while. Get used to that then try skimmed again or just stick with semi if you can't take that next step.

Cutting down on snacks between meals is an on going battle. Perhaps I was really meant to be a grazing animal. Eating healthier snacks might be a good way to go on this as so far I haven't had much success in giving up this habit.

Sugar is a problem for me. I enjoy sweet foods and I have dealt with this by avoiding foods with a high sugar content because I found that the more sugary food I ate the more I craved. Sugar is addictive for some of us. I believe that experiments performed on rats show that rats will choose sugar over normal food and even over cocaine! The rats will continue to eat sugar long after they have had sufficient calories and long after rats on normal food will stop eating. The sugar seems to override their normal instincts. You can see this to some extent with people too. Very few people refuse dessert even if they have had trouble finishing their main course. It seems there is always room for sugar. I have managed this fondness for sweet food by giving up desserts except for special occasions or if the dessert is fresh fruit. If I am eating in a restaurant I am not usually tempted by the sweet trolley as experience has shown me that although the food looks tempting it is all in the eye and not in the taste. I will have a starter instead as I don't usually have the full three courses.

As I am eating less sugar I am finding that I want less. Eating sour foods does seem to re-educate your taste buds so you find very sweet foods quite sickly and cloying. Is anyone out there old enough to remember the lemon juice diet? Drinking a glass of lemon juice and water was supposed to help you lose weight by decreasing you appetite for sweet things. If I remember rightly it did seem to help but I really disliked the lemon juice so the diet didn't last long. If I eat too much sweet food the craving for more kicks in so it is easier just to cut sweet foods down to a minimum.

You get sugars from the fruit you eat and from some vegetables like carrots and if I'm not eating concentrated sugar I enjoy these things more.

Don't let friends persuade you that it's OK to use honey as a sugar substitute. It has just as many calories and it is just as fattening. It may (or may not) have the many other miraculous properties that they claim but being low calorie is not one of them.

Watch out for hidden fats and sugars in processed food. Fat and sugar are cheap ingredients so manufacturers are keen to use a high proportion of them in their products. They turn up in surprising amounts in canned soup, baked beans, sauces for pasta or curry and all sorts of other unexpected places. "Low fat" often means high sugar as the manufacturer tries to make the product more appealing. I try to read the ingredients list on the label and to only use these items occasionally if I am tired or in a hurry. Otherwise I make my own sauces and thicken with cornflour rather than making a roux using butter. When you check the ingredients remember that all those that end in "ose" are in fact all sugars e.g. dextrose. glucose etc. Listing these separately helps to disguise the total amount of sugar contained in the item.

I avoid too many obviously high fat foods like pastry, sausages, doughnuts, fried food etc. I am sure you could add lots to the list. Most snack type foods are high in fat. I do eat butter as I loathe all the nasty substitute spreads and I eat a lot of cheese. A point to remember is that fat is fat and has the calories even if it is olive oil. Olive oil might be better for you than lard but it still has the high calorie count of other fats.

This is the way I have become used to choosing food over the last few years. I am flexible but these are the general factors I consider when I'm shopping in the supermarket or eating in a restaurant. I have jars of sauce and tins of soup in my store cupboard for use in moments of crisis or idleness but I try not to use these things on a regular basis. I think I'm now much more aware of what is in the food we eat and so I can make more informed choices.

Having put in the effort of fasting I am reluctant to throw away the weight loss benefit so I still watch what I eat in between times without being obsessive or counting calories. The single most important thing I have done is cut down on portion size. If your family are big eaters too then maybe you could do this together?

Chapter 7. Exercise... or not?

The diet does not demand that you exercise.

However exercise does improve your muscle tone.

The choice is yours.

I have found that I feel so much better on this diet that I want to be more active. I feel much more at home in my own body so I enjoy getting out in the fresh air and walking. For me walking has a number of benefits that are not related to diet and weight loss but that enhance my life. I find that a walk helps me to think and to resolve problems. It helps me to put things in perspective if I am angry or upset. I notice the changing seasons, the sky and clouds, the changing colours and reflections in the water. This adds to the richness of life. Of course I am lucky to live in a place where there are a variety of pleasant places to walk. Often I can fit a walk into my daily life by walking into the village to go to the shop or the doctors' surgery instead of taking the car. Meeting other people and keeping in touch with village life is another bonus of being on foot rather than driving.

I have always been resistant to any form of exercise that requires special clothing. I just don't want the bother of getting changed so, although I quite like swimming and know that it's good for you, I very seldom go to the pool. (Maybe people in warmer climates feel differently about this?) Walking is one of the few things that doesn't require any special equipment or clothing so it is easy for me to just walk out through the door.

I have to admit that I have had very little exercise lately but I have still lost weight. The weather has been so wet for the last few months that there hasn't been the opportunity to get out much. I have reached an age where I prefer not to set out in heavy rain. I don't mind if it starts to rain while I am out but I don't set off in a downpour without a very pressing reason.

In conclusion while I think exercise is optional on this diet it does have benefits that it would be a shame to miss out on.

Chapter 8. In the end...

What will I do when I reach my target size?

I will have a big celebration and also buy some new clothes!

My target at the moment is to fit comfortably into a UK size 16 (US 14, EU 42). When I have reached that goal I will still want the health benefits of the fast diet. I plan to move to just one fast day each week and to buy some bathroom scales. I plan to actually use the scales and if I start to put on weight I will just go back to two days fasting each week for a while.

I think it will take me about another 12 to 18 months to achieve this but I feel sure that I **will** be able to carry on with this way of eating until I do - and afterwards.

I feel so much better, mentally and physically already, and I hope you find the same benefits if you decide to give it a try. It has been well worth the effort and a very positive experience so far. It really is working for me.

Acknowledgements

Dr Michael Mosley whose television programme I watched.

He has recently published a book and I have a copy on order now. In case you want all the information straight from the horses mouth here are the details:

The Fast Diet by Dr Michael Mosley and Mimi Spencer

I have discovered this book is available on the web after ordering from a bookshop so you will not need the catalogue number - which is a good thing as I don't have it to hand!

Related books from the publisher:

Other diets you may be interested in:
Blood Type Diet;
http://www.amazon.com/dp/B008YTM5JS
Mediterranean Diet Exposed;
http://www.amazon.com/dp/B009H8RQ6C